I0090511

TOP
FITNESS
ADVICE

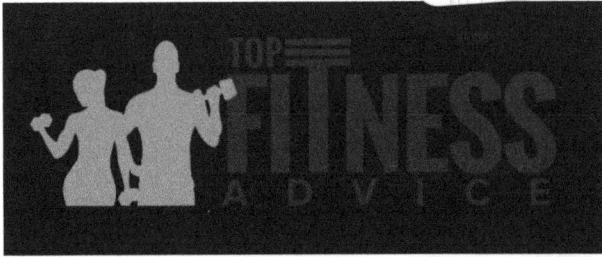

EMOTIONAL EATING

How To End Emotional Eating, Get Healthy & Finally Free Yourself So You Can Be Happy

Kayla Bates

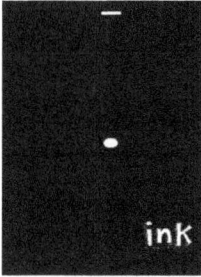

First published in 2017 by Venture Ink Publishing

Copyright © Top Fitness Advice 2019

All rights reserved.

No part of this book may be reproduced in any form without permission in writing from the author. No part of this publication may be reproduced or transmitted in any form or by any means, mechanic, electronic, photocopying, recording, by any storage or retrieval system, or transmitted by email without the permission in writing from the author and publisher.

Requests to the publisher for permission should be addressed to publishing@ventureink.co

For more information about the contents of this book or questions to the author, please contact Kayla Bates at kayla@topfitnessadvice.com

Disclaimer

This book provides wellness management information in an informative and educational manner only, with information that is general in nature and that is not specific to you, the reader. The contents of this book are intended to assist you and other readers in your personal wellness efforts. Consult your physician regarding the applicability of any information provided in this book to you.

Nothing in this book should be construed as personal advice or diagnosis, and must not be used in this manner. The information provided about conditions is general in nature. This information does not cover all possible uses, actions, precautions, side-effects, or interactions of medicines, or medical procedures. The information in this book should not be considered as complete and does not cover all diseases, ailments, physical conditions, or their treatment.

You should consult with your physician before beginning any exercise, weight loss, or health care program. This book should not be used in place of a call or visit to a competent health-care professional. You should consult a health care professional before adopting any of the suggestions in this book or before drawing inferences from it.

Any decision regarding treatment and medication for your condition should be made with the advice and consultation of a qualified health care professional. If you have, or suspect you have, a health-care problem, then you should immediately contact a qualified health care professional for treatment.

No Warranties: The author and publisher don't guarantee or warrant the quality, accuracy, completeness, timeliness, appropriateness or suitability of the information in this book, or of any product or services referenced in this book.

The information in this book is provided on an "as is" basis and the author and publisher make no representations or warranties of any kind with respect to this information. This book may contain inaccuracies, typographical errors, or other errors.

Liability Disclaimer: The publisher, author, and other parties involved in the creation, production, provision of information, or delivery of this book specifically disclaim any responsibility, and shall not be held liable for any damages, claims, injuries, losses, liabilities, costs, or obligations including any direct, indirect, special, incidental, or consequences damages (collectively known as "Damages") whatsoever and howsoever caused, arising out of, or in connection with the use or misuse of the site and the information contained within it, whether such Damages arise in contract, tort, negligence, equity, statute law, or by way of other legal theory.

Table of Contents

Would you prefer to listen to my book, rather than read it?

Download the audiobook version for free!

If you go to the special link below and sign up to Audible as a new customer, you can get the audiobook version of my book completely free.

emotional
eating

How to **End Emotional Eating,**
Get Healthy & Finally Free Yourself
So You Can Be Happy

kayla bates

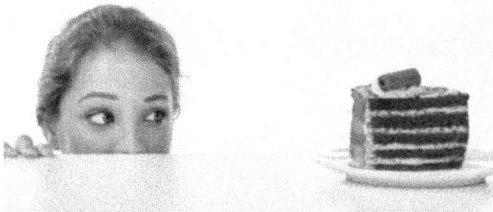

Go here to get your audiobook version for free:

TopFitnessAdvice.com/go/EmotionalEating

Introduction

First off, congratulations on deciding to make the effort towards building a healthier and more positive stress-free life. Change is never an easy thing, but once you set the wheels in motion, you're going to want to continue to stick with your new way of life free of stress and the emotional eating that comes along with it.

When it comes to living a stress-free life void of emotional eating, don't forget that above all else, stick with that road your on in achieving it. Don't give up. Anything is possible if you believe in yourself, have an awareness of what's going on with your mind and body, and want to make that change from being burdened with too much stress and coping with binge eating to living a life where you can proudly say stress doesn't run your life anymore.

By being aware and making the changes, not only are you making a statement for yourself, but you are giving motivation to others who may be experiencing the same types of stress related issues that have been plaguing you. Here are a few last tips to help you maintain your newfound, healthy lifestyle:

Don't forget to smile! Especially when it means being proud of yourself for overcoming the stress in your life and taking control of your emotional eating. Smile, laugh, play, and just enjoy your life free from stress. Not only is it a positive way to keep a stress-free lifestyle, but it's contagious as well. You're sure to brighten someone else's day and perhaps even encourage them to not sweat the everyday stresses in life.

Enjoy daily meals with your family: Not only is this essential to maintain a healthy relationship with your family members, but it's also a conscious way to make sure help manage your stress and avoid falling into an emotional eating trigger.

Always get a good night's rest: Getting enough sleep is always essential for a healthy lifestyle. And when you wake up feeling rested and refreshed, you're going to be less likely to worry about any stressors that you may encounter that day.

Stay positive: Having a positive attitude is one of the best ways to maintain a healthy, stress-free lifestyle. Don't let the small things get you down. Embrace them and face them head on. You'll find that with a positive attitude, anything is possible.

Lastly, don't forget that it's okay to falter every once in a while. You are human after all, and we are all going to make mistakes. The beauty of making mistakes is what we learn from them.

Don't forget to record those mistakes in your stress journal! In time, you'll be able to look back on those mistakes as a positive reminder of how far you've come. Just remember, in the grand scheme of things, there's always going to be some kind of stress to face in your life. It's how you address it, face it, and handle it that makes all the difference!

Thanks for purchasing this book. It's my firm belief that it will provide you with all the answers to your questions.

What is Emotional Eating?

Everyone has experienced emotional eating at some point in their lives.

If you have ever eaten a favorite food when feeling sad, worried, stressed out, or as a reward for achieving an accomplishment or celebration, then you have experienced emotional eating. Emotional eating is eating to satisfy an emotional need rather than a natural hunger.

Using food occasionally in this way is not a bad thing. It is only troublesome when you repeatedly reach for food to soothe your feelings.

Food is just a temporary relief but does not cure the emotional problem. When overeating continues, so do the feelings of guilt and shame as you gain extra weight and feel more and more out of control.

Not sure if you are an emotional eater? Take the emotional eating test below:

Emotional Eating Checklist

- Do I eat food even when I'm not hungry?
- Do I eat food to feel better such as when I'm bored, angry, sad, worried?
- Do I feel food has control over me?
- Do I eat more food when I'm feeling stressed?
- Do I usually eat until I feel stuffed?

- Do I reward myself with food?
- Do I see food as a friend?

If you answered yes to 2 or 3 of the above questions, then this book is for you!

Emotional Hunger or Natural Hunger?

It is important to recognize the differences between emotional hunger and natural hunger before you can be mindful of your emotional eating habits. There are five main differences:

- Emotional hunger strikes suddenly and feels urgent. Natural hunger comes on gradually with no real urgency to eat immediately.

- Emotional hunger is brain hunger. It involves craving specific foods that are sweet, salty or fatty and there is a feeling of needing to eat the food now. Natural hunger originates in the stomach as a pang of hunger. Any food will do, including healthy foods.

- Emotional hunger involves mindless eating when you can eat a carton of ice cream without realizing it. Natural hunger involves being more aware of what you are eating as you concentrate on satisfying the hunger.

- Emotional hunger often leads to self-loathing, regret or guilt because you know in your heart that you are not eating for nutritional needs. When satisfying natural hunger, there is no need to feel ashamed because you know you are giving your body what it needs.

- Emotional hunger has no sense of satiety. You feel the need to eat more and more food until you are uncomfortably full. With natural hunger, you can stop eating when your stomach is full and feel satisfied.

Are You ALWAYS Hungry When You Try to Lose Weight?

Discover How to STOP Starving Yourself & Lose Weight FASTER By Eating MORE Food!

For this month only, you can get Kayla's best-selling & most popular book absolutely free – *The Ultimate Guide to Healthy Eating & Losing Weight Without Starving Yourself!*

Get Your FREE Copy Here:

TopFitnessAdvice.com/Book

Discover how you can **start eating MORE food** and see weight loss results faster than ever before. Learn about the 10 most powerful fat-burning foods and how they boost the rate that your body burns fat. And last but not least, finally put an end to your emotional or "bored" eating habits. With this book, readers were able to significantly improve their weight loss results. So, it's highly recommended that you get this book, especially while it's free!

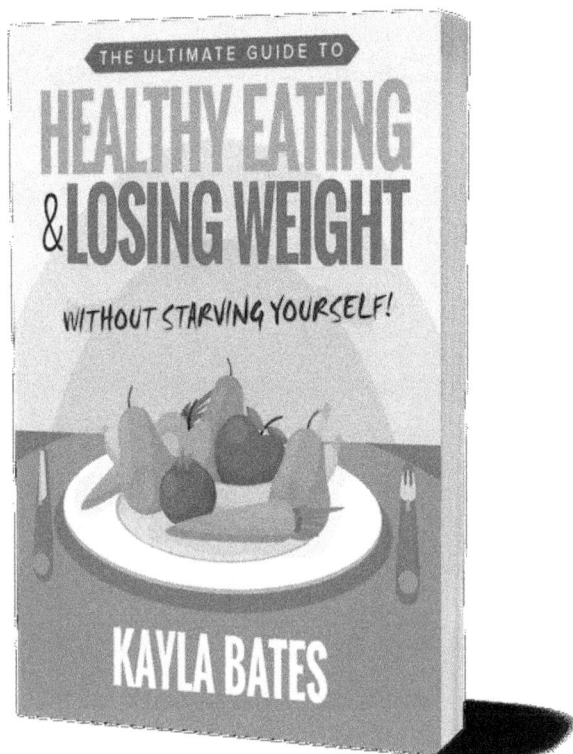

Get Your FREE Copy Here:

TopFitnessAdvice.com/Book

Causes and Symptoms of Emotional Eating

Emotional Eating is defined as the process in which someone consumes a large amount of food, usually food that is unhealthy such as "junk foods," so that they could somehow feel better.

In short, people afflicted with Emotional Eating Disorder use food as a means to alleviate the pain or loneliness that they are feeling.

You may not be aware of it, but you or people you know may have Emotional Eating Disorder, too. It's not hard to be afflicted with the disorder because almost everyone knows that food is something that's easy to get, and somehow, people think that over-eating or comfort eating would not do anything wrong with their bodies, since, after all, we all need food to live.

However, one should know that comfort eating will do some distress to our bodies. Depression, guilt, anxiety, chronic frustration, stress are some of the things that one could experience once he/she gets in the throes of emotional eating.

One may also be afflicted with diseases or ailments such as Diabetes, High Blood Pressure, Obesity, Malnutrition, Depression, Anxiety, Menstrual and Digestive Problems.

So, how does one know that he/she is afflicted with emotional eating or if his/her family members of friends are afflicted with the said disorder? Here's what you should know.

Common Triggers of Emotional Eating:

Many things/situations can be considered as causes of Emotional Eating. These are the following:

- Emotional, or when someone eats because of feelings of loneliness, pain, fatigued, stress, anxiety or even boredom. When someone feels like he/she has no idea how to let out all the bad feelings that have taken over his/her life, then this person may want to eat just to fill the emptiness that he/she has been feeling.

  Sometimes, when people feel good after eating, they tend to think of it as a way that will help them get over sadness and pain, and that's why they tend to eat more than they could handle, even if they are not even hungry, at all.

  Sometimes, a person also feels happier or feels a sense of joy after eating a lot and thus, this person thinks that he/she is doing the right thing. Sometimes, people also turn to food when they are going through a break-up, or grieving over a death in the family.

- Mental, or when someone thinks that he/she is not good enough; when someone feels pressured about something; when someone thinks that he or she is not being appreciated; or when someone just seems to be so troubled that he/she feels out of his/her wits.

- Situational, or when one eats because he/she is watching something on the television; is looking at a movie; is in a restaurant or fast food chain and is compelled to order more than what he/she really is capable of eating; eating too much junk food when watching sports, or watching a game; eating while being parked in front of the computer all day, etc.

- Social, or being compelled to eat because other people are around; eating at parties or gatherings;

  Incidentally, this also means that one may eat when he/she is not comfortable in social situations, or when he/she feels like he/she does not belong in the place where he is situated.

- Physiological, or when someone skipped meals and feels very hungry so he/she may eat more than he/she may handle; when someone wants to eat because he/she is not feeling well, etc.

As you may notice, the things written in here are pretty much normal situations. However, what makes them wrong is the fact that when someone overeats due to these situations/causes, then it means that person is afflicted with Emotional Eating Disorder.

Remember, even if we all need to eat to live, you have to remember that eating too much is not good. Too much of anything is never too good at all.

Here are the common symptoms or signs of someone who has Emotional Eating Disorder:

- Over-eating when in a stressful or painful situation. For example, if someone gets scolded at work, has too much work to do, or has problems with friends/family or relationships.

- Eating too much and consecutively in a short period.

- Eating until one feels stomach or even emotional pain, or eating until one feels like throwing up.

- Being unable to control the amount of what someone is eating.

- Feeling ashamed or guilty after one of your binges.

- Getting back to this habit all the time.

If you think that you or someone you know exhibits these symptoms, then it's time that you let go and break free from your Emotional Eating Disorder and start living a better, healthier life.

I hope that you are enjoying this book so far, and if you could spare 30 seconds, I would greatly appreciate you leaving a review on Amazon.com.

Trap Those Triggers

It's difficult to stop a problem that you can't see. If you don't recognize the triggers that cause you to crave food, it's like swatting at invisible flies. You might get it right someday, but it'll save you a lot of time and effort if you make yourself aware of the feelings that stimulate emotional eating.

Be honest: it isn't a shameful thing to want to be better. You will only be doing a disservice to yourself if you don't conduct an honest self-assessment. Take a look at the ten most common triggers of emotional eating:

Stress

Signs: You have to work late for the umpteenth time in a row. You could have sworn that you've been at it all day, but the paperwork on your desk doesn't look like it lessened an inch.

The work that needs to be finished would normally take half a day, but the deadline is in an hour and your hopes of getting promoted lie in the success of this project.

Maybe you lose hope and reach for your nearest comfort food, or you convince yourself that eating a chocolate bar would give you the energy you need to finish this. Either way, you have an urgent meeting with a sugary treat.

What You Crave: Stress isn't something to be taken lightly. People these days are conditioned to accept that stress is a regular part of life, but it shouldn't be. It might be difficult to handle the level of work you receive every day, but you can deal with it by finding a way to de-stress.

Instead of reaching for a donut, do a bit of exercise at your desk. If you know how to meditate, that's a great way to release stress as well. Remember that overeating can lead to weight gain and health problems, so don't add to your stress by being an emotional eater!

Loneliness

Signs: Another weekend is here but you have nowhere to go or no one to go with. Maybe you just went through a rough break-up. Maybe you've been noticing how your group of friends has been drifting apart for the past few months.

The bottom line is you feel you're all alone, and it stinks! You can feel something is missing in your life, so you fill it up with fatty or sugary food. It makes you feel better, and that's all that matters.

What You Crave: This is an obvious one, you might think. And it is. Everyone needs a bit of physical companionship. That doesn't mean you won't be able to feel happy without it. Many people currently in relationships long for the freedom of being single.

If you want a new friend or significant other, then make the first move. Join a class you're interested in taking, or maybe try looking online. Don't wait for them to come to you. Be proactive!

Low Self-Esteem

Signs: You avoid looking at yourself in the mirror. When you do, an overwhelming feeling of disgust or shame takes over. You hate something (or everything) about yourself, and you feel that nothing can change that.

What You Crave: If you feel bad about yourself for being a certain way, then overeating can be like a form of punishment. You may think that you deserve to feel terrible about yourself, but the opposite is true. As soon as you wake up, think of one thing that you or someone you know likes about yourself. No one is perfect, so be proud of what makes you human.

Anxiety

Signs: You tend to bite your nails or run your fingers through your hair constantly. You're familiar with that feeling of time being both too slow and too fast all at once.

Whether it's the little things or major life-changing events that keep you up at night, you know that one thing that gets you feeling better is a bite (or two, or three) of cake or chocolate.

What You Crave: Close your eyes and take a deep breath. You may not be able to control whether a certain event happens or not, but you can control the cravings you get.

If it's something like an important presentation for work that makes your fingers itch for a bag of chips, then choose to grab an apple or other fruit instead.

Social Situations

Signs: It's your weekly lunch date with your friends, and you just know you'll be eating more than you want to. You can't help it! It's not like they're forcing you to eat; you just feel that it would be awkward if you just stared at them while they're getting lunch.

Maybe you're afraid they'd call you out on it if you ate too little. Another case is when you don't even know that you're eating too much because you're too focused on talking and catching up with friends.

What You Crave: They're your friends. If they won't be able to understand your choice to stay away from emotional eating, then who will? Always be conscious of what you're doing when there's food around you.

Don't overdo it, though. If you're complaining to your friends about how miserable you feel over eating a single French fry, then that's not good either. Aim for a healthy moderation.

Anger

Signs: It was that guy who cut you off in traffic who caused all this. You just want to put your head out the window and scream at him, but he's gone now, so what do you do? You feel like you have to do something. Anything.

So, you yell at someone else or maybe eat a muffin or two to calm down. Even mild cases can cause you to overeat, like being annoyed at a co-worker or being frustrated with yourself for not being able to complete a task.

"If I had anger issues, I'm sure someone would have told me," is a common response from people who are asked if they get irrational feelings of anger. What they don't realize is that, in most cases, people don't call them out because they're too afraid of riling them up.

If yelling at your family, writing mean and anonymous comments about your boss, or eating fattening foods is your way of expressing anger, then this is your trigger.

What You Crave: You need to release your tension healthily. Don't suppress or hide it by stuffing your anger with food. Eating may calm you down, but it shouldn't be your go-to solution when you're angry.

You can play relaxing music or try focusing on an audio book instead. Those who want to get physical can go for a sport like boxing or maybe run around the track.

Boredom

Signs: There are days when nothing is good enough to hold your interest. The TV remote's barely in your grip anymore, and you could swear you've seen this show at least three times before. There's nothing to read or watch or listen to. Even lying down isn't good enough.

During these times, food seems like a great solution. It's yummy, it makes you feel something, and you feel good for a change! Bad news, though: that's not real hunger. If you keep that habit up, it'll eventually lead to weight problems and more.

What You Crave: Imagine how vast the world you live in is. You can't even begin to imagine all the experiences you haven't tried yet. There's no reason to be bored. You just haven't found the right activity to stimulate you mentally.

Get out of the house. Make it your goal to find a way to distract yourself for ten minutes. By the time your alarm sounds off, your cravings would have passed. Engage your mind!

Happiness

Signs: There's no day like today! You've got a great, big smile on your face, and you feel like nothing can get you down.

It could be because of a promotion or a compliment from a special someone. Whatever it is, you know that a slice of pizza would make you feel even better!

What You Crave: Everyone wants to be happy. Once you are, you never want to stop. Eating sugary food can maintain those good feelings temporarily, but they come with a hefty price tag. You might feel a sugar crash take away the happiness that could have been there longer if you didn't indulge in your cravings.

If you're happy and want to stay that way, then do something fun, preferably outside. Take a long walk or visit a friend. The sun would surely be shining on you no matter what!

Depression

Signs: It's that restless feeling you get when you're convinced that everything you do is meaningless. Though serious depression should immediately be brought to a therapist, having a case of the blues is a common reason for people to eat. They want to feel the warmth of a sugar rush.

What You Crave: Maybe you haven't seen sunlight for days. Maybe you've had a string of bad luck lately, and you feel like the whole world is against you.

Ask a friend to take a walk with you and tell them what you're feeling. The exercise will boost your serotonin levels, and talking to a trusted friend will ease some of the weight on your shoulders.

Just Because You Can

Signs: It's that time of day again. You take out that tub of ice cream—your favorite flavor for years—and make your way to your favorite chair. It's practically a tradition.

What You Crave: It's a bad habit you need to break. Every person needs habits to go through their daily life with ease. When it's a bad habit, it keeps you shackled to the same old routines. You think that you can't make it through the day if you don't give in to that craving.

Try to do something different at least once. Take note of it. Try to do a different thing tomorrow. Be conscious that you were able to change your tradition without anything bad happening. Believe in yourself!

There are several more triggers that could cause you to reach for the nearest sugary treat. Triggers like physical pain, frustration and fear also exist.

If whatever you're feeling results in a craving, then that's a trigger for you. Write that down immediately so you can make a tally of the times it happens. You might be surprised at how often a specific trigger can cause you to eat when you're not hungry.

Setting Yourself Up for Success

There is, unfortunately, no one-size-fits-all nutrition program that we can all agree to follow for ultimate health and a perfect body.

We all have different needs when it comes to the ideal nutritional outline. Things like activity level, weight loss goals, taste buds, diabetes needs, gluten allergies, lactose intolerance, or choices like veganism, and what truly fits into our lives makes our needs different than our friends'.

Developing your new relationship with food takes time. You will learn how to expect that you just might fall "off the wagon," and how to get back on that wagon quickly.

In this chapter, you'll learn how to acknowledge personal progress in your evolving relationship with food. Believe it or not, the hardest part of your progress might be giving you credit for making progress!

In the past, when you've tried to assess your progress, you may have been rather hard on yourself. Too hard on yourself. You may have demanded perfection, and forgotten that you're human, and it takes a time to change something immense in your life.

Yes, some theories say it takes 30 days to create a new habit, but you're not simply changing an action in your life—you're studying yourself and learning about your relationship with food. If you spend the next five years continuously evolving the choices you make around food, consider that incredible progress.

Your relationship with food is always evolving. What works for you this year might not fit in your life next year. Remind yourself, it takes time, and you're making progress day by day.

Let's begin with what happens when we feel like we've taken a step back, skip over the part where we beat ourselves up for it, and learn how to get back on track:

Falling "Off the Wagon" & Getting Back On that Wagon Quickly

Chances are, you will not go your entire life without overeating or emotionally binging ever again, even if you've gone weeks or months without a relapse.

The difference between any future binges and your binges of the past lies in your ability to pick yourself up, dust yourself off, and get back on track.

Whether you fall off the wagon for one evening or two whole weeks, don't linger there with guilt.

The moment you choose to acknowledge what you're doing and decide that you'd like to stop, is the moment you launch your personal "Pick-up Plan."

Your "Pick-up Plan" consists of 3 steps:

- **Acknowledge what happened:** Write down or share with a friend exactly what led you to use food as an emotional outlet. Be as specific and honest as you can. Get it out. Acknowledge the truth. Turn towards it.

- **Immediately forgive yourself:** There is no room in your plan for guilt, shame, or self-blame. Instead, you will quickly and truly forgive yourself for abusing food. Write it down. Look at yourself in the mirror and forgive yourself for being human.

- **Focus on Your "Pick-Up Phrase":** Your "Pick-up Phrase" is a short sentence that helps you re-focus on your personal goals for your health and your relationship with food. Example: "I will feed my body with compassion and respect."

Millions of people embark on new diet plans to whip into enviable shape, but the majority of them fail early. To increase your chances of success, use these simple tips for dieting effectively and harmlessly.

Set realistic goals

If your expectations are too high while dieting, your attempt is more likely to result in failure. It is crucial to set reasonable goals for your diet to avoid disappointment, so don't expect to lose twenty pounds in a week. Losing anywhere from three to five pounds a week is considered a healthy amount of weight loss.

Track your progress

If you want to ensure that your diet is working, you must track your progress. A weight loss notebook can be used to chart the amount of weight that you lose each week, the types of exercise you did, and the duration of each workout.

Also, keep a food diary of everything that you eat, the amount eaten, and the time that you ate it. You may find that a certain combination of foods and exercise is quite effective.

Use technology to your advantage to assist you as well. Try a fitness app on your Smartphone or tablet to help you record your progress.

Go for fresh foods

Fresh foods are better for your diet plans and your system. Sugar and salt add unhealthy weight quickly, and they are hidden in canned and frozen foods. Select fresh foods whenever possible for preparing each dish. Buying your healthy food in bulk encourages you to eat healthier, and it also saves you money.

Use portion sizes

Many folks mistakenly over-eat because they are not aware of the proper portion sizes at mealtime. Most portion sizes at restaurants and even when one prepares food at home are strikingly off.

Keep in mind that your stomach is only about the size of a fist, so avoid stuffing yourself. Make sure that every meal is divided into three portions: ¼ lean meat, ½ vegetables, and ¼ a starch of your choice. Use smaller plates to avoid stocking up.

Don't rush your meal

Eating too quickly does not give you time to feel full. As a result, it often leads dieters to overeat. Take your time to chew your food carefully during every meal to better monitor your eating. Drink water while you eat to limit consumption.

Take vitamins

If you feel like your energy is zapped, then you are more likely to return to your normal eating patterns in an attempt to feel better.

You can avoid backsliding into your old eating habits by taking vitamins daily to improve your basic energy levels and bodily functions.

Avoid skipping meals

Responsible, healthy eating is the best way to lose weight naturally. Skipping meals is the worst thing a dieter can do.

Starving yourself even messes up your metabolism, and it makes it much harder for you to lose weight. Eat three times a day to maintain the nutrition levels needed for a healthy body.

Get enough rest

If you want to have enough energy to succeed in dieting, you need to get enough sleep every night. Your body uses sleep to repair itself, and it gives your body time to adjust. Aim for eight hours of rest every night, and go to bed early.

Cut back on emotional eating

Addressing the causes of emotional eating is essential if you want to achieve your target goals. Periods of stress and anxiety are more likely to arouse emotional eating in both men and women, so relieve your stress daily.

Learn how to identify when you are hungry, or if emotional ups and downs spark your craving. Beware of binging on junk foods, processed products, and other poor selections to avoid sabotaging your diet plans.

Motivate yourself

If you want to succeed I any diet, you will have to rely on self-motivation during times of temptation and weakness. Put pictures up of yourself as you lose weight in areas that you will see them so that you can admire your progress.

Make a vision board of all the desirable things that you will wear or do once you lose the weight. As you see the pounds slide off, you will gain more motivation to propel you towards your goal.

Work with a friend

One way to set you up for permanent weight loss success is to work together with a friend. A friend or a family member who has fitness goals themselves can be a phenomenal influence in keeping you on the right dietary track.

Exercise regularly

Any diet plan gets a strong boost when it is used in combination with an exercise regimen. Exercising vigorously for at least 30 minutes a day does weight-loss wonders.

Start by walking or jogging for 20 minutes a day, and work your way up. Switching up your exercises with cycling, swimming, yoga, and aerobic challenges your body and encourages the continual shedding of pounds.

Join a local gym

It is easier to stay on track if you commit to going to a local gym. Visiting a gym two or three times a week is a great incentive to stay on your diet. Consider hiring a personal trainer to guild you in developing the bets body imaginable. A personal trainer can help you work on problem areas with targeted exercises to lose weight much faster while you are dieting.

Make small improvements

It can be daunting to go on a full-fledged diet plan right away, so ease yourself into the process. Start by incorporating more leafy greens and fruits into your daily diet, and you will find it easier to persevere long-term.

Do not crash diet

Going on a crazy crash diet is bound to set you up for failure. You may lose some weight at first, but it often comes back with a vengeance after the diet is over. Also, a wild crash diet can lead you to the emergency room. Utilize only logical, healthy dietary plans to lose the fat and keep it off your figure.

Stick to your dietary goals with fervor, and make the changes necessary to win the weight war. Following these dietary tips will ensure that your present weight loss goals shift into reality.

Once again, thank you for reading this book, and I hope you're getting a lot of valuable information. I would greatly appreciate it if you could take 30 seconds to leave me a review for this book on Amazon.com.

Enjoying this book?

Check out my other best sellers!

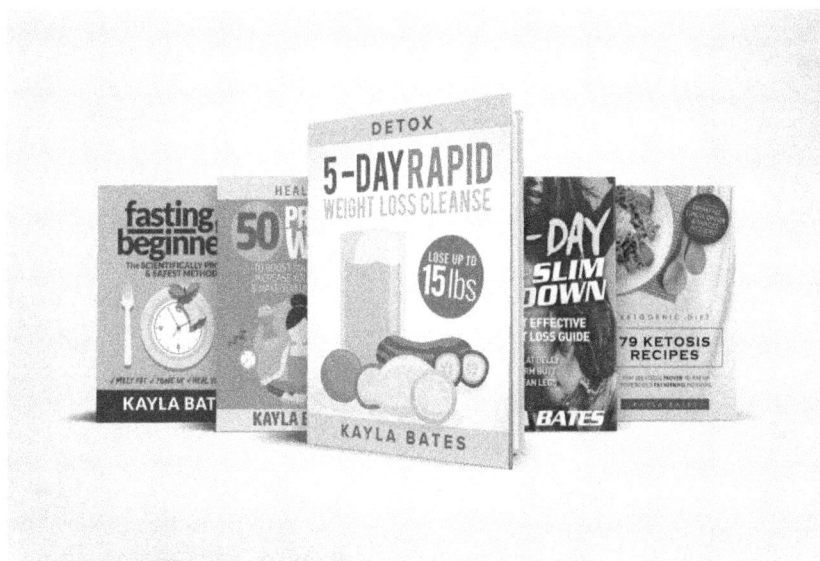

Get your next book on sale here:

TopFitnessAdvice.com/go/Kayla

How Do You Stay Slim and Eat What You Want?

Contrary to popular belief, it is possible to eat what you want and still stay slim while doing so.

This is not to say that it is at all easy, though. It requires unwavering focus, commitment, and effort not only from you but also from those around you—your significant other, family, friends and other people with whom you maintain close contact. You will have to be disciplined about your diet and exercise regimen, both of which will be key to your success.

The simplest way to eat what you want and maintain your trim figure is to substitute out certain common foods and cooking ingredients when you are preparing your meals and snacks. This may sound like restrictive advice, but you will be amazed at how creative you can be with food when you put your mind to it.

Palate-pleasing, waist-expanding ingredients such as butter, sugar, white flour, milk chocolate, salt, pre-made sauces and marinades, alcohol and high-calorie drinks will either need to be eliminated from your diet altogether or only consumed sparingly.

If you can be good 90 percent of the time, indulging during the other ten percent will not derail your efforts to stay slim and trim. Now, without further ado, here are some tips to follow if you want to eat what you enjoy while keeping the pounds off:

Use Substitutes in Your Cooking

As discussed above, this is essential. Substitute olive oil or pureed avocado for butter, honey or Stevia for sugar, oat flour for white flour (all that is required to make oat flour is some oats, a blender or food processor and a couple of minutes of your time), dark chocolate for milk chocolate, powders and herbs for salt, black coffee and unsweetened tea for high-calorie drinks such as soda and fruit juice, diet tonic water for high-calorie mixers used in cocktails and neat or on-the-rocks liquor (sparingly, of course) for beer or white wine.

The occasional indulgence is permissible but should not become a habit if you want to continue seeing positive results.

Find an Exercise Plan That Works and, Most Importantly, Stick to It

There is no one-size-fits-all exercise and fitness plan. It is up to you to know yourself and what will help you achieve your goal. Running, spinning, yoga, CrossFit, weightlifting, recreational sports and even walking your dog are all solid workout options for minimizing the size of your waistline. Find something that is effective and enjoyable to

Learn to Control Your Portions

As the saying goes, your eyes are often larger than your stomach. Pace yourself while you eat, and try eating with smaller plates or bowls. People have a tendency to measure their food intake by the plateful or bowlful, so minimizing the size of these dishes will do wonders to keep you in check.

Finally, wait until 20 minutes after you have finished your meal to eat dessert. More often than not, you will find that you are no longer hungry and that you saved yourself from consuming excess empty calories.

Eat Several Small Meals Rather Than Two or Three Large Ones

Eating throughout the day means your digestive track is likely not getting much of a break. This works in your favor, as digesting food requires the body to expend energy. Yes, your body is burning calories without you even realizing it.

The alternative is the feast-and-famine experience your body goes through when it is only being fueled two or three times per day, which leads to a few bursts of digestive action and much longer periods of uninterrupted inactivity.

These periods of inactivity result in less work for your digestive system, which means that you are not expending energy and burning calories.

Eat Breakfast Like a King, Lunch Like a Commoner and Dinner Like a Pauper

Yes, you should be eating more than three meals per day. That is no excuse for following the spirit of this saying, though. Your food consumption should be highest in the morning and lowest at night, with the middle of the day falling somewhere in between the two.

Try to eat your carbohydrates—almost all of which should be complex, by the way—in the morning. This is a great time to eat some oatmeal, which is cheap and extremely easy to prepare, along with some foods that are high in protein and good fat such as eggs (or if you are so inclined egg whites), low-fat Greek yogurt and nuts or nut butter. The best evening and night choices are rich in good fat and protein.

Believe in Yourself

No matter how hokey or hackneyed it may sound, you have to believe in yourself. Failing to do so will be a huge detriment to your success.

Skills of Developing Healthy Eating

The best way to follow your meal plan is to choose the food that goes well with your snacks. This means the food you take should feel you comfortable to eat and should not lead you to binge eating.

In the early stages, you would think of taking a low-calorie food or diet food. But this is not a problem since you are trying to move away from the idea of eating to control your weight. This way, you should easily come out of the vicious cycle of dieting and bingeing.

Don't think that you will increase a lot of weight with this diet; instead, try to think that this food will make you healthier and stronger. When you change your aim from losing weight to becoming healthier, than the food you want the most is the food that makes you feel best.

What you eat at each meal can affect your energy levels and moods. Keeping a food diary should help you to recognize your eating patterns. All the information that you need will be available to you to help you determine the changes you need to take in your meal plan.

If you think that it's hard for you to recognize your eating patterns, then you can consult your dietician or nutritionist for the best suggestion. Monitor your blood sugar levels time to time to understand any metabolic changes in your body due to your meal plan.

Create benchmarks in your meals to control your eating habits. Planning meals and snacks in advance are the best way in this case. Another effective way is to decide how much you are going to eat in a single meal and put only that much amount of food on your plate.

Choose one food as your "food stopper," e.g. choose a piece any fruit like orange as your food stopper and end your meal with it. This ensures that your meal has a pre-planned end and you should not put yourself to bingeing this way.

I have seen that many people make a stockpile of food products at their kitchen, but this is not plausible in case you are following a meal plan.

Planning your meal in advance should also help you to shop more mindfully for your food, and you must not overstock foods that tempt you to binge. Try your best strategies to support your efforts to take back control and use them to your advantage.

Many studies have proved that the smell and looks of your food can encourage you to eat a healthy meal. So, try to make every meal as appetizing and attractive as possible. You can celebrate the meal by lighting candles and music.

When you use all your senses to take your meal, you should increase your awareness and attentiveness that keeps you mindful of what you are doing.

Try to avoid any distractions during your meal like TV, newspaper, mobile, or computer. Rushing your meal is often counterproductive, and your main aim should be mindful eating.

Try your best to stick to the decisions you have made. If you feel hungry even after you have finished your meal, then try to ignore this feeling and stick to your decision not to eat anymore.

Adapt your plan for the following day and try to learn from your experiences. Reviewing your food diary at the end of each day will help you to achieve your goal.

Others who are considering purchasing this book would love to know what you think. If you could spare a few seconds, they would greatly appreciate reading an honest review from you. Simply visit the page on Amazon.com.

How to Ensure the Eating Disorder Never Comes Back

1. Create a healthy environment

How do you change your environment when dealing with a problem that is more or less compulsive in nature?

Well, you work like a mathematician: from the known to the unknown. Right now, you can identify the environment that overwhelms you into eating in an unorthodox manner. So, the same way a plant dies when you deprive it of water, you are going to work at dismantling the structures that facilitate the bad environment.

If, for example, every time you go out drinking with your spouse you must have a bitter argument in return, getting a different pastime other than drinking will be the first step. That way, you will not find yourself sitting on the couch the following day sulking and eating.

If you stopped working only because your spouse wanted you to be a housewife, and now you are feeling all miserable, address that fact with your spouse.

Once you get back working and life becomes more interesting to you, the joy will be felt in your household, and your relationship will be stronger. Such a healthy environment has no room for emotional eating.

2. Love yourself

Be your benchmark. There is nobody else like you in this whole wide world. Even when you are a model on the catwalk, remember there were many other girls where you came from yet they never made the cut.

Incidentally, when you meet them today, they may have less money than you do, but they do sincerely look happy. Do you not realize then, that any time you spend worrying about how people perceive your body is time wasted? Would you have died if you had not made it to the catwalk? No – of course not.

Possibly modeling was not even your first career choice but other people looked at you and gave you the idea. It is time you started to appreciate yourself and just live a normal life. Try to eat like you did when they found you, a humble, lanky but healthy girl.

The changes of the glamorous lifestyle are the ones that are doing you in; like eating out almost always instead of eating home-made food. Or living in limousines and elevators when not on the catwalk as you are now too important to go anywhere on foot. Suppose you then scheduled work-out hours and kept to them – no more and no less than scheduled?

In fact, it would do you a lot of good to keep in touch with some of your old friends because they will keep reminding you how lucky you are to be you.

3. Seek to counsel on pertinent issues

You may find that you do not want to miss the drinking you have so much been accustomed to, even though you know that the routine is to argue with your spouse after that and then eat yourself to sleep.

In that case, you might, very likely, have developed a drinking problem, only you have not given it much thought. You need to have a session with a psychologist or other professional counselor, who will assess your situation and help you design a helpful roadmap to healthy eating.

Remind yourself that this kind of eating is responsible for your weight spiraling out of control and your heart rate is a concern to your doctor. Make a flashback when life was so much fun, and you will have something to look forward to. In fact, you might wish to speak to your spouse about couples' counseling.

If the company you have worked for in the last 10yrs is restructuring and laying unrealistic demands on the skeleton workforce left, you might want to consider applying for other jobs elsewhere. Do not let your sense of loyalty to the company numb your sense of happy living.

Essentially, the wish to be happy never really goes away; it is only veiled in other ways like overeating or overdrinking.

4. Structure your life

Have a clear daily plan, where you break down your activities regarding hours. Allocate leisure activities to free time so that you will not have to yawn at some point and wonder what to do next.

Included in this structuring should be a meal plan. You need to know what is on the menu as you get to each day. In fact, it is helpful to have the menu in an open place, possibly in the kitchen, as that makes every family member his or her 'brother's keeper.'

It will be a challenge, for instance, for your kids to ask why you are eating off the biscuit packet early in the morning when there are wheat flakes on the breakfast menu. That kind of challenge will keep you on the straight and narrow, eliminating casual and careless snacking.

5. Stock healthy foods

Sugary foods and those that are deep fried and salted, have a way of keeping your palate asking for more. So, instead of having those in the house, you could stock foods that, though delicious, are complex in nature and are not so sweet.

These are foods like bran flakes; wheat flakes; fibrous fruits; vegetable salads; and such other delicious but satisfying foods. Those will come in handy when you have real hunger and will not encourage you to keep eating once you are full.

6. Do some exercise

Exercising, albeit for a few minutes each day, has a way of releasing 'happy hormones', with neurotransmitters that make you feel happy and positive about life.

Besides, when you exercise, you get tired and have no time to worry about things that do not matter. You will not, for example, have time to think what your colleagues think about you not getting a promotion or you getting a divorce.

When you exercise, you get tired, take a shower, replenish your spent energy with some food that you very well deserve, and after that, you enjoy your relaxation. And when you go to bed, you sleep like a baby.

7. Reward yourself for goals achieved

It is important to have a target of things you want to achieve. For every step you progress, give yourself a specific reward with a definite time frame. That way, you will be happy with your life because you are making progress.

If you have set your reward as a weekend get-away, for example, you need not worry about overeating during that time as you have a specified time limit. That leeway you give yourself will also make you not miss any food on a daily basis, the way you do when you label the food taboo.

8. Keep the company of positive people and people with a purpose

When you visualize happy people, it is unlikely you see people buried in the kitchen all day long eating or people pitched on bar stools drinking themselves silly all day.

To the contrary, you possibly see a crowd of fans cheering their sports team on; a group of people dancing their feet sore in a reward party after completing a challenging project. Sometimes you see innocent kids running about playing excitedly without a care in the world.

Whereas you are not a child who has no idea the world has its rough edges, you, can allow yourself some fun. Just sitting down and watching a nice movie is a healthy way to relax and give you a healthy laugh.

Also, when your friends have projects underway, it is unlikely you will be the idler in the circle of friends. You will find yourself thinking of ideas to benefit your family and the community around you.

Whatever you do whose results are fulfilling once you are through, will make you happy and your life meaningful. Happy, busy people do not binge.

Why You Have Failed in the Past

Diets Fail Because of Out of Control Emotional Decisions

Calorie Controlled Diets don't work on a permanent basis – for you or anyone else. Of course, eventually you'll have to embrace a lifestyle where you enjoy eating delicious, healthy food and a fun and regular exercise routine, but first, you must focus on what specifically makes you feel helpless in your life, especially about eating food.

You may be feeling more optimistic at this stage, but I suspect that you're also skeptical and may even harbor doubts about ultimate success. Your gut may be saying to you, "Can something as intense and as strong as my emotional eating needs be changed?"

This Program is going to help you understand things about yourself that you may have tried to hide or conceal and when you realize and accept these things about yourself, you will finally understand that you don't need to let food and eating control and ruin your life.

We are going to give you a mirror to reflect your behaviors, motivations, and all of the habits that are not serving you well. Emotional overeating is destructive to your health and happiness – your focus will finally be on you and not your food.

But this place of self-doubt is the starting point where everyone who needs to change emotional eating habits has to begin their voyage of transformation and empowerment. Once you get past the old habits of skepticism, we'll be ready to look at why you have been stuck in the same downward spiral for so long.

The multi-billion pound/dollar Weight Loss Industry assumes that because you're desperate to lose weight, you'll have enough positive intention to stick to any weight-loss program and succeed. And that might work for a little while at least.

As you've discovered, eating generates immediate comfort and rewards, whereas the rewards you get from staying on a controlled diet won't be noticeable for weeks or maybe even for months.

Future possible benefits versus the immediate desire for a tasty mouthful or two - or three! - That's the well-charted recipe for yo-yo dieting. Positive motivation alone simply can't overcome the addictive desire for the immediate taste sensation that propels you to eat the things you know you shouldn't. That's so obvious now.

Food Encourages Your Feelings of Helplessness

We talked about how eating takes you to your early emotional development, predominantly because as infant's food was often associated with nurture, comfort, and love. However, childhood is also associated with helplessness. As a child, you were, in fact, petty much helpless. You were dependent on others to love, protect and nurture you.

Although food provides you with some of the nurturing comforts of childhood by taking you back to that state of mind, when you use food this way, you're reverting to a childish way of dealing with the world. And that reminds you of the helpless feeling of being a child. It's a vicious circle.

But you're an adult now and you have real adult choices: you can be in charge of the powerful destiny of your life by facing your emotions and listening to what they have to say to you, or you can continue overeating to cope with negative and scary emotions, knowing that it actually keeps you stuck in childhood, a place where you were in fact helpless.

Confronting your emotions makes you an adult, the only place where you have the possibility to experience what it's like to be powerful finally.

For emotional eaters like yourself, you often can't see the woods for the trees. In the moment when emotions have been triggered and the helplessness reaction kicks in, eating in a certain way feels like a life-or-death decision.

When you distract your inner turmoil with food, it's not a handful of berries or nuts. It tends to be bigger than normal quantities of food, typically unhealthy foods, and the foods are eaten in a voracious, aggressive way – more like chomping and swallowing without tasting rather than eating with awareness.

By the time the emotional eating frenzy has ended, the scary negative feelings have vanished, but they have not disappeared. They're just somewhere under that huge mound of food, almost like lost documents on a hard drive – they exist somewhere but are temporarily unavailable. You're more addicted to the reprieve that the food provides than to the food itself.

I hope you have learned something from this book so far and would greatly appreciate it if you could leave an honest review on Amazon.com.

Asking for Help

If you are still feeling like you cannot do this, make sure to ask a professional for help. Find the right friends and family members who will support you and push you to keep going. Right now, you can't afford for people to just coddle you along in this journey.

You do not have to do this alone even though you may feel alone. There are other alternatives out there: Paid professionals that can help you identify the sources of your stress or make it clear what your goals are in life.

You will find some excellent support groups. Choose one that is within the area and attend their sessions. Talking to and sharing ideas and experiences with people who are in the same position as you is a great way to verbally express yourself.

Writing your feelings is one step, and saying them out loud is another. There is something very powerful that happens when you share your feelings with a group. It is like you are hearing your own story for the first time and finally understand it. You can pick up additional tips, techniques and strategies that might work for you also in these groups.

When you pick the group, you will still need to be mindful of the people who are surrounding you. If you are only complaining about your disorder but not taking action to improve, you need to find a different group.

Preferably the group will have some people in it who have successfully defeated their eating disorder. They can be a wealth of information and can really help you along your journey. Make sure to fully utilize your journal to record everything you are feeling and learning.

An effective program for eating disorders should be able to address the very symptoms and triggering factors of the disorder. It is not enough just to temporarily alleviate the symptoms: If the root cause of the problem is not addressed, then it will just be a cycle that will happen over and over.

If you are going to see a doctor, here are some therapy treatments they may recommend:

Cognitive-Behavioral Therapy

This treatment focuses on the behaviors and thoughts a patient associates with binge eating and/or overeating. The purpose of Cognitive-Behavioral Therapy is to make you aware of how you use food in dealing with emotional changes. You will be able to establish what triggers cause you to binge eat or overeat so you can avoid them. The treatment includes nutrition education, relaxation techniques, and a weight loss program.

Dialectical Behavior Therapy

This one fuses together mindfulness and Cognitive-Behavioral Therapy techniques. The main purpose of this treatment is to help you to accept yourself as a person to avoid negativity. It also teaches you to manage stress better and keep your emotions in check.

Interpersonal Psychotherapy

This focuses on your interpersonal issues that have caused you to overeat or binge eat. Your therapist will teach you how to communicate your feelings better so you can build a more solid relationship with your loved ones and the people around you. This treatment will help you deal with your emotions when you encounter relationship problems.

As I close this chapter, I just want to reinforce the fact that you do not have to do this alone. Sharing your emotions and pain with someone can seem like a daunting task, but it is forever uplifting. Have a good cry or make it a good full out sobbing session. Whatever releases it from your system so you can clear the way for recovery.

A good cry never hurt anyone, and it might take more than one along the way to keep progressing. Contrary to popular belief, crying is not a sign of weakness; it is a sign of strength, the type of strength needed to let go and to not be consumed by negativity.

Whatever path you choose to take, ensure you find the support you need.

Other Things to Remember

Here are other things that you have to keep in mind to beat your Emotional Eating Disorder:

- Three full meals a day, or 5 to 6 small meals a day is considered healthy. Anything less or more than that would put your health in peril.

- Eat a healthy breakfast. As they say, breakfast is the most important meal of the day. Once you eat a good kind of breakfast, then your mood for the day would be good, and you would stop being too emotional or too inclined to eating even when you shouldn't be.

- Eat a heavy lunch. Of course, if you're at school or work, you need something that will keep you up and would add up to your energy and enthusiasm for the whole day.

  It's also important to eat lunch because sometimes when one skips this meal, it may be a cause or trigger of someone developing Emotional Eating Disorder.

  A good kind of lunch is something that is rich in protein, and those that are made from lean products. Here are some examples:

- Eat a light but fulfilling dinner. Yes, the body's metabolism is very slow at night, and that's why it's important to eat something light, but also to make sure that this something light would be able to compensate for all the nutrients that the body needs.

Eat healthy snacks:

- Sliced tomatoes with olive oil and Feta.

- Air-popped popcorn.

- Fruit or vegetable juice with no added sugar.

- Milkshakes made from skimmed milk.

- Dried fruit.

- Granola bars or trail mixes. These are great because they are a combination of fruits and nuts and are nice to snack on. Plus, you will not gain an ounce of fat from them.

- Canned fruit, such as Lychees, Peaches, or Mangoes.

- Fruits such as Strawberries or Cantaloupes.

- Raw baby carrot sticks. You seriously would not realize that time is passing as you eat this healthy snack.

- Turkey Jerky. It's healthy, it's filling, and it's the kind of snack that you can just munch on whenever you feel like you need something to munch on.

Remember, the key to being healthy is remembering that you have to keep some sense of balance in life, especially when it comes to your diet.

Once you learn how to keep your diet balanced and healthy, then you would be able to avoid eating when you are not feeling well or having some emotional issues in life.

Learn how to spot the triggers. Learn what pushes you to over-eat and try not to get so affected anymore. Remember, there are so many things that you can do with your time. Focus on that.

- Get enough sleep. Sometimes, you make a hasty decision or feel so much stress because you haven't been sleeping well. Get at least 6 to 8 hours of sleep each night.

- Control your brain. You own your brain, and your brain does not own you. Remember that and learn how to enjoy new things, form new habits and focus on what you could still change your life for the better.

- Make a list of goals that you plan to accomplish. Divide this into short-term and long-term goals and make sure that you get to accomplish something, no matter how little it may seem.

  You could write something as simple as "I will no longer eat potato chips five times a day," or "I promise to enroll in class"—whatever it may be, it's okay. What matters is that it is something that would help you become a better person and that you'll learn to let go of your emotional eating addiction in the long run.

- Do not be too hard on yourself. Remember that we all have flaws, and we all have imperfections, but it does not mean that we are not worthy of anything. You are an important person and you were created for something good. Remember that.

- Throw away the scale. Throw away the weighing scale. It does not mean that you are just going to let yourself go; it means that you will strive to be healthy and you would not allow unnecessary pressure from yourself or from the world to rule your life. It's time for you to be healthy from this day forward.

- Focus on the now. Your past may haunt you and may be your reason for over-eating, but remember that you still have today, tomorrow and your whole life to make up for it. You can still make new memories. And, you can get over your emotional eating disorder starting today.

Don't forget to share your thoughts on this book by leaving a review on Amazon.com. It takes just a few seconds.

Are You ALWAYS Hungry When You Try to Lose Weight?

Discover How to STOP Starving Yourself & Lose Weight FASTER By Eating MORE Food!

For this month only, you can get Kayla's best-selling & most popular book absolutely free – *The Ultimate Guide to Healthy Eating & Losing Weight Without Starving Yourself!*

Get Your FREE Copy Here:
TopFitnessAdvice.com/Book

Discover how you can **start eating MORE food** and see weight loss results faster than ever before. Learn about the 10 most powerful fat-burning foods and how they boost the rate that your body burns fat. And last but not least, finally put an end to your emotional or "bored" eating habits. With this book, readers were able to significantly improve their weight loss results. So, it's highly recommended that you get this book, especially while it's free!

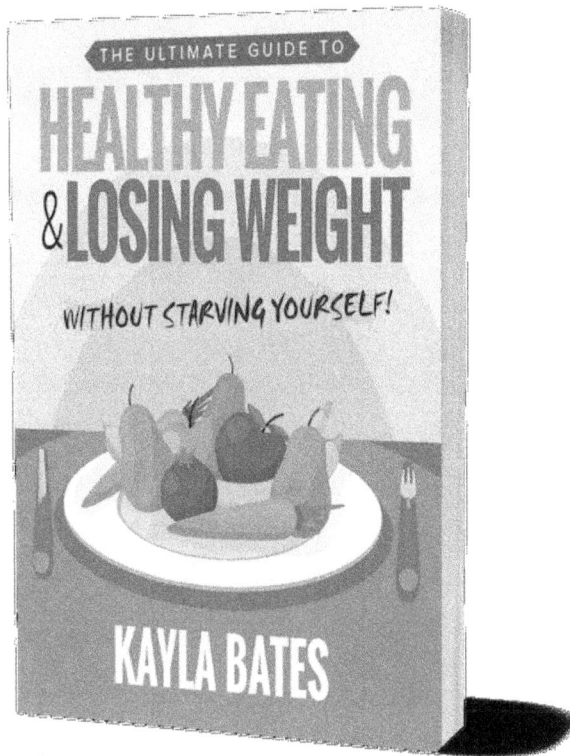

THE ULTIMATE GUIDE TO

HEALTHY EATING
&LOSING WEIGHT

WITHOUT STARVING YOURSELF!

KAYLA BATES

Get Your FREE Copy Here:

TopFitnessAdvice.com/Book

Conclusion

Change is upon you and the quality of your life is about to improve. I would wish you luck on your journey, but there is no such thing as luck: There are only the people who choose to take action and confront their eating disorders or don't.

Sure, the people who recover from an eating disorder seem lucky, but it all came down to them choosing to be different, to do something new and make a change for the better.

I am proud of you for reading this book. I hope my unique approach will allow you to be free from your overeating. Your motivation and commitment will come from you really wanting to do this.

I can talk all I want, but until something clicks inside you that says now is the time to change, there is little else I can do.

Thank you for taking the time to read this book. This is your body, your choice and your life. Never forget you always have the power to choose how you live that life. I hope I was able to help you gain control of your eating habits.

Enjoying this book?

Check out my other best sellers!

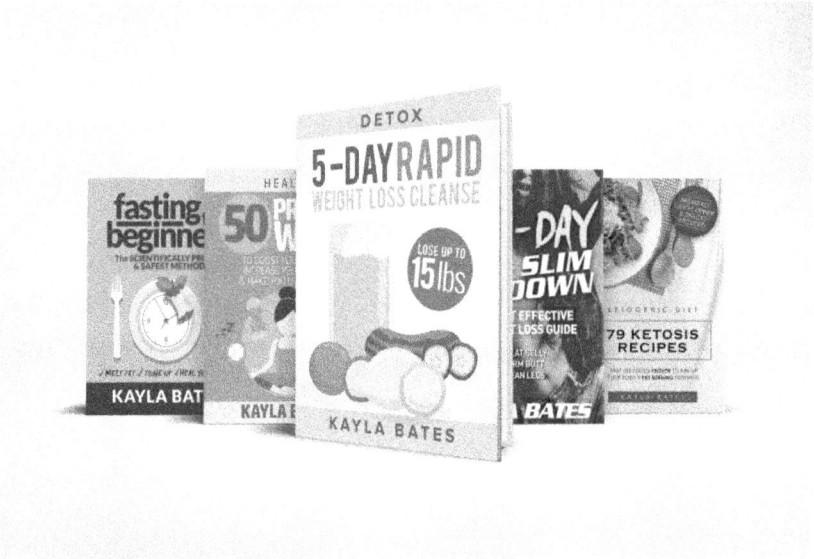

Get your next book on sale here:

TopFitnessAdvice.com/go/Kayla

Final Words

I would like to thank you for purchasing my book and I hope I have been able to help you and educate you on something new.

If you have enjoyed this book and would like to share your positive thoughts, could you please take 30 seconds of your time to go back and give me a review on my Amazon book page.

I greatly appreciate seeing these reviews because it helps me share my hard work.

You can leave me a review on Amazon.com.

Again, thank you and I wish you all the best!

www.ingramcontent.com/pod-product-compliance
Lightning Source LLC
Chambersburg PA
CBHW031209020426
42333CB00013B/857